Saturday Night Knife & Gun Club

by L.S. Collison

Episode #2

Kit Carson's Knife and Gun Club

America's New Wild West

Cover design by M.G. Manelis
ISBN: 978-7322290-0-6 (paperback)
ISBN: 978-0-9893653-9-0 (electronic edition)
Copyright © 2018 by Linda Collison
Fiction House, Ltd
Steamboat Springs, Colorado

continued from...

Friday Night Knife & Gun Club

by L.S. Collison

Saturday Night

Kit Carson, RN

In my dream the bad guy was trying to kill me. I couldn't make out his face, but I knew he was the bad guy because of his black hat. In my dream, I drew my gun, but it came out of the holster reluctantly. I was moving sooo slooooooow. I took aim just below the black hat. Now the bad guy's face was materializing out of the shadows, it was coming into focus, illuminated by a golden light from above. I squeezed the trigger. In my dream the face became Wyatt's. He looked at me sorrowfully in that last instant before the bullet found its mark.

*

I awoke in a cold sweat. Wyatt, shaking my shoulder impatiently, Calamity's plaintive voice whining like a gnat in my ear.

"Mommy, wake up, pleeeease? We're hungry. There's nothing left to eat."

I buried my head under the pillow and mumbled, "Grab some money out of my saddle bags. Go buy Pop Tarts or something."

"Mom," Wyatt said in a stern and strangely adult voice. "Wake up. The money's all gone."

Get a grip, my conscience chided in agreement. *You're out of work, out of money –you're in deep shit, woman.*

*

After the Friday night shooting spree, the hospital had given us the boot – every last one of us --and High Plains Medical Center shut its doors. *Wild West Today,* dubbed it "The High Plains Massacre," but ten days later another shoot-out snatched the headlines, and we became just another notch in the ragged holster of American history.

Another few days, maybe a week, and the recent shootings were completely forgotten in the nightmare of the upcoming election. Bully Ratzer was promising to "Make the West Wild Again," while the incumbent, Marjorie Bledsoe, whose voice was shrill as a schoolmarm, wanted to overturn the Guns-for-All Guarantee and the Chinese Exclusion Act. I honestly didn't care who won, I just wanted it to be over.

In a futile attempt to disarm the nightmares, I had spent the days and weeks following the hospital shooting (now down-graded from a Category 4 Massacre) in a self-medicated, whiskey-and-weed induced torpor. I hadn't gone to my friend's memorial service, I hadn't gone to the candlelight vigil held for the victims, and I

6

had failed the Emergency Sharpshooter Response course required for my nursing recertification. My kids had been expelled from school for truancy and I didn't even know it, so shit-faced was I.

*

It was Tonto who rescued me. Tim Rhodes, that is; the former TICU charge nurse at High Plains Medical Center. Tonto got us both per-diem gigs – temporary work at the medical center across town. Wellmart. Night shift, Emergency Department. I was desperate enough to do anything – even Emergency. Even night shift. Even Wellmart.

Rhodes was the quiet, self-assured type. Proud of his Indian ancestry, he wore moccasins and kept his long hair, gray at the temples, in a braid. Tonto and I had worked together for three years, yet we hardly knew each other outside of the trauma unit, and I wondered why he hooked me up with the gig when he might have asked any number of unemployed nurses.

*

Our first shift was a Saturday night. The Indian and I were thrown in cold. There was no orientation for hired guns like us. A busy charge nurse pointed to the crash carts and the medication dispensers, issued our access codes, then threw us to the wolves. Of course, as temp nurses, Tonto and I were given the shit patients.

Standard procedure. But we dealt with it, uncomplainingly. To tell you the truth, it was nice to be working again.

*

Hospitals aren't that different, one from the next, and Emergency Rooms work pretty much the same all across the West. People love to complain about ERs. Give them a chance and they always relate horror stories, mostly about how long they had to wait and how nothing was done for them. Yet the fact that they came out alive says something. You don't go to the ER for a shave and a haircut.

My first patient of the night was Cindy, a thirty-six- year old barmaid at the Wrangler Saloon. Cindy came in with a sudden onset of lower right quadrant abdominal pain. I knew right away this would be a long work-up because abdominal pain is a mixed bag. It can be caused by an obstruction, a GI bleed, an ectopic pregnancy; it can be appendicitis, a pulled muscle, peritonitis, PID, or plain old gas.

The doctor was busy in the next room trying to save the life and larynx of a twelve-year-old who had accepted a social media sword-swallowing challenge (with the expected result). Knowing Doc would be tied up awhile, I drew Cindy's blood and collected a urine sample and sent them off to the lab. Then I got my first drunk of the night, apparently one of the regular customers; he knew all the other nurses by name. This was more or less a babysitting assignment, but drunks can get into trouble in the ER. They can fall and break their neck, they aspirate on their own vomit, they can even die on you.

It had been several years since I had worked in the Knife & Gun Club, a.k.a. Emergency Department, Emergency Room, or ER as it has been long referred to as. But I knew what I was in for. ERs are situations of controlled chaos, especially on the night shift.

Working ER is kind of like playing a game. A sick game. Here's how it's played: Patients come in randomly and the object is to get rid of them – either admit them to the hospital or send them home – as quickly as possible. You get extra points (and better social media reviews) if you keep them alive and relieve their suffering while giving them a "positive customer experience." In the ER, we use wits and skills to defeat the opponent. But unlike a game, when Death scores in the ER, there aren't any time-outs or replays. After twenty or thirty minutes of coding a pulseless patient, when the Doc looks at the clock and calls it, the game's over.

The deaths of strangers stay with you like a chronic, low-grade infection. Each loss of life affects you deeply, maybe even on a cellular level. But you don't even realize it at the time. You're just trying to keep the fuckers alive and satisfied. You're just trying to send them home.

Enough morbid philosophy. I was glad for the gig; I'd be making good money here. No bennies – but who needs PTO or health insurance? Retirement? Fuck it; pensions are for snowflakes. If you can't stand the heat, get out of the kitchen. It's high stakes in this poker game and winner takes all. Me? I'm struggling right now, but hey, I've got my rights. Not healthcare rights, not reproductive rights, not education rights – but I've got my gun rights. A Gatling gun in every home – let's make the West wild again.

*

"You're new around these parts," the ER doc said, handing me a chart. She squinted against the garish florescent lights, sizing me up.

"Kit Carson, RN," I said. "I'm a hired gun. I work for the Agency."

"Ruth Halliday," she said, touching the brim of her slouch hat. "Are you Mr. Barker's nurse?"

I nodded.

"He needs blood gasses."

"It's as good as done," I said. Actually, it *was* done. I had already drawn them and sent them to the lab, anticipating the order. Doc's the head honcho, but in Emergency we work as a team.

Doctor Ruth Halliday was a scowling, taciturn woman in worn-down boots and leather chaps that had seen some hard riding. She was an old buffalo soldier, I could see, from the medal-of- honor on her vest. I would grow to trust her and respect her, if not exactly like her. Halliday knew her shit, she could rope, ride, and brand with the best. She knew how to keep those ponies rollin', rollin'. Like the old ER doc's ballad goes,

Move 'em on, head 'em up

Head 'em in, cut 'em out

Get 'em out of my ER,

Rawhide!

Send 'em to the floor

Kick 'em out the door

Come morning we'll be living high and wide...

*

Half past midnight, I needed to pee, but the stampede was on: We were swamped with Saturday night bar fights, knife fights and random shootings. In came the broken bones and kidney stones; chest pains and migraines, common colds and psychiatric holds, overdoses and halitosis -- all seeking refuge and relief inside

Wellmart's hallowed halls. No time to eat, no time to piss, but we were gittin' 'er

done. Setting bones, suturing wounds, sedating psychotics.

It wasn't until quarter past four in the morning that we finally got a little

breather. (Note: Nurses never say the "Q" word while on duty. *Ever.* To utter the

word Q-U-I-E-T is bad luck and guarantees that all hell will break loose. It's one of

the first things a brand new nurse learns when she starts her first job.)

Zero Four-Thirty. My drunk was tucked in and sleeping soundly, his bag of

yellow nearly finished infusing. I was restocking my rooms when Tonto appeared

with a cup of coffee in hand. Smelled good, too, burnt though it was.

"You got a minute?" he said.

I knew what he meant—a little break on the ambulance ramp where we could get

our nicotine fix. My heart did a little skip and jump, like a girl playing hopscotch.

I've always thought Tonto was kind of hot. For an older guy, that is. Yeah, I had a

minute. Maybe more.

*

I bundled up in my duster and neckerchief, my hat pulled down against the biting

wind. Tonto slipped a motorcycle jacket on over his scrubs, tied a bandana tied

around his head. We stood outside the ambulance entrance sharing the coffee,

passing the Marlboro between us.

"What do you ride?" I asked.

"A Sportster," he said.

"I hear you're badass with a bow and arrow," I said. "Is that true?"

He shrugged. "Come to the archery range with me sometime and you can make up your own mind." Tonto had a reputation with a bow and arrow, but I knew nothing at all about Tim Rhodes, the man behind the myth. In the hospital, everybody's got a nickname, a persona, an avatar. Mine's Kit Carson. We don't put our real shit on our badges in case some patient or family member decides to get a little too friendly and stalk us. Or has a vendetta against us.

"So how are you holding up, Kit?" Tonto spoke quietly, his voice, matter-of-fact. But I knew what he was getting at; he was poking at my vulnerable spot, probing that festering wound. My best friend had been killed in the hospital shooting, accidentally shot by one of the other nurses.

I didn't answer. Tonto took a drink of coffee, passed me the cup. The simple gesture made my eyes sting.

"You okay?"

"I'm alive," I quipped. I didn't want Tonto or anybody else see me cry. *Toughen up, buttercup.*

"Yeah, me too," he said. "We're both alive. We should make the most of it."

Suddenly desire surfaced like a joker in the deck of cards that were my emotions. A roll in the hay with Tonto might be just what I needed.

But that too passed. We made small talk—the weather, the news. I wanted to talk about things that mattered. The meaning of time and the universe. My feelings. My hopes and dreams. Neh. Couldn't bring myself to do it. So much easier to repeat slogans and sound-bites. To talk like we text, in smiley faces and emojis.

I drew the last of the cigarette and crushed it out on the icy pavement under the heel of my boot. The wail of a train whistle passing through town cut through my soul. Hearing that sound always made me wish I was on that train, any train, heading somewhere, anywhere. I glanced at my watch; it was time to go back inside and finish the shift.

Tim passed me the last swig of coffee, cold now. I drank it like I was dying of thirst.

Nearby, the sound of squealing tires. Suddenly, there it was – a black livery hauling ass up the ramp. Oh shit; looks like trouble.

The car screeched to a halt, the rear door opened and a body tumbled out onto the pavement at our feet. A bruised and beaten body, unconscious and entirely naked but for the tassel on her left nipple. The car didn't wait but instead drove off, the rear door still open.

"Back to work, kemosabe," Tonto said.

Down on our knees we went.

"No breath, no pulse," I said, fumbling for my pocket mask. Being closest to her head, I got the airway. Tonto, already astride her torso, his stacked palms on her sternum, two fingers-width up from the xiphoid process, right between those magnificent silicone breasts.

"Hell's bells, it's Stormy Wether," said Tonto, sucking in his breath.

"You *know* her?" I said, then blew into the pocket mask. Her chest rose and fell compliantly.

He shot me a look as he pumped, circulating my breaths through her body. "Are you kidding me? Every man in town knows Stormy Wether. Or at least knows *of* her. She's renowned for her choreography."

"Her choreography?"

"She's a dancer down at the O.K. Corral." Tonto finished the cycle of chest compressions and paused while I gave the celebrity two more breaths.

The O.K. Corral was the kind of establishment most women didn't go to, unless they worked there. Although I was told a woman owned it.

"Is she gonna make it?" I heard a young voice say.

15

I looked up to see a scantily-dressed girl standing nearby, hugging herself for warmth. She had long bare legs, a knife tucked snugly into a garter belt high on her left thigh. Cheap flashy spurs on fuck-me boots.

"Please save my sister," the girl said, her teeth chattering. "She's all I've got in the world."

Tonto called a code on his phone, and within ninety seconds flat we had all the sharpshooters out on the ramp. Doc Halliday and the A Team to the rescue. A respiratory therapist with a bag valve mask relieved me of my duties; Tonto continued with compressions. We got Ms. Wether on a backboard, through the doors and into Trauma Room #1.

"V-tach, 150. No pulse."

"Let's get some saline going. Type and cross for two units. What's the story?"

"I've got 14-gauge in. Running normal saline, wide open."

"Arrived unconscious, signs of trauma to head and thorax. Possibly assault with a blunt object."

"Continue chest compressions. Hyperventilate and stand by with suction, please. Get me a curved blade and a 7.5 ET tube, let's get her tubed."

"Portable X-Ray standing by."

The entire team worked together following ACLS protocol. It was a beautiful thing to behold.

*

The girl who called herself sister had followed us in and was peeking around the curtain. Her face was badly bruised. I know a fist to the face when I see one. I took her into the adjoining room and pulled the blue curtain closed.

"What's your name, honey?"

"Balmy," she says.

"Barmy?"

"Balmy," she corrected. "Balmy Wether. It's my stage name; I'm a dancer."

Stormy and Balmy Wether. Clever branding, you've got to admit.

"Have you seen me on social media? I've got over five thousand followers on my channel."

"Balmy, that pretty face of yours took quite a punch. Let me have a look."

"I'll be fine," she said, turning away. "It's my sister I'm worried about."

I got her a cold gel pack from the refrigerator, wrapped it in a washcloth. "Here, put this on your eye, it'll help." She flinched when I touched her. "Now then, tell me what happened tonight."

She removed the gel pack to look at me from behind a dark curtain of bangs. Oh, those eyes, those puffy, purple eyes! I assured her the swelling would go down and the bruising would fade, but I wondered to myself if the youthful light would ever return or if she could even remember her innocence.

I had danced for a man, once. My ex. Did a couple of suggestive moves holding onto the poster of our conjugal bed. He had asked me to and I obliged him, feeling rather silly. I remember how excited he had become, the power I seemed to have over him at that moment. Men are strange creatures; normally strong but weak when it comes to their desires.

Balmy wiped a trickle of blood from her upper lip with her finger. "They came into our dressing room after the show. After the bar closed down."

"Look, honey," I said. "We should call the law. Whoever did this to you, they need to be caught and punished."

"No." She was adamant. "You can't do that."

"Why? Are you in some sort of trouble?"

"Yeah," she said with a dry laugh. "You could say that. My whole life has been trouble. But if you call the dawgs my sister is dead, I'm dead, we're both dead."

My skin tingled hearing the calm certainty in her voice.

"How old are you, Balmy?"

"Twenty," she said.

"You mean sixteen?" I countered.

"I'm old enough to know what men want and how to give it to them," she huffed, hand on hip.

My eyes stung with a burst of sympathy for her. I remembered myself at that age—half child, half woman. "Look, Balmy, I'm on your side. My name's Kit. I'm a nurse; I've got your back."

She met my eyes and we had a pact.

"So tell me more about what happened. Who were these men, do you know?"

"Bully Ratzer's guys."

"*Sheriff* Ratzer?"

She nodded.

"You're telling me Sheriff Ratzer assaulted you?"

Her eye roll said *Duh*, like only a teenager can. "Not Ratzer himself. His thugs. You know, his posse?"

"Why?"

She snorted, impatiently. "Why do you think?"

"At your age you should be babysitting and barrel racing," I said. "Junior Rodeo. Have you thought of joining the Westernaires? The Prairie Scouts?"

She stuck her bottom lip out in a sullen pout. "Don't be so parental."

"I don't mean to be. I can't help it. I've got kids of my own."

"Besides, I make good money performing. Stormy says we'll be real movie stars one day."

I felt disheartened even though she probably made more money than I did. "How much—never mind, don't tell me. The money's not important. Tell me what happened."

"Ratzer's a good customer. A real good customer. Stormy had a special thing going with him, but a few months ago he gave Stormy an envelope of cash; I saw it myself. And he had her sign an agreement, some legal document, and she promised to never say a word about what went on between her and Bully. For a couple of weeks, we were living large. Room service, new clothes, a trip to San Francisco. Then the money ran out and Stormy said it wasn't right to keep silent. On account of Ratzer running for governor. She said the people have a right to know the truth about him and that piece of paper she signed wasn't worth a damn."

"Sit down and let me have a look at your face. You could have a fractured orbital bone. We should at least do an X-ray. And that laceration on your chin, that could use some stiches."

"No," she said. "I don't want my name in the records. I've got to get out of here, find someplace to hide."

"But you're underage. And you're the victim of abuse. I'm obligated to report that."

"You call the law, nurse, and I'm dead."

"Look, I'll do everything I can to protect you. You're safe here in the hospital."

But the girl knew better than I did. "No. I'm not. They're here, Ratzer's goons are here, they followed us."

"Here?" I drew my piece and looked around warily.

"Hey, what's with the gun?" she demanded. "I thought nurses and doctors were supposed to save people, not shoot them. What about the Hippocratic oath?"

"Well, it's complicated," I said. "We have to protect ourselves and our patients. This is the Wild West, you know?"

"I don't buy that."

I put the pistol back in its holster. "So how many of them are there?"

"Two men, maybe three. I don't remember, not clearly. They had masks on. Two of them have thick, hairy arms and little peckers. I bit one of them on his wrist and drew blood."

"You saw their genitals?"

She blinked slowly. "In my line of work, I see a lot of them."

"Yeah, me too."

"Well, I guess we've got that in common," she said. Her smile was a flash of tiny pearls.

"My sister, she's going to be OK, isn't she?"

Just then my phone buzzed, alerting me to a new patient. I pulled it out of my pocket and read the text to see what I was getting. An S.O.B. (that's shortness-of-breath, not son-of-a-bitch)—and when I looked up, Balmy was gone. *Vamoose.* Nowhere to be seen.

*

I started to assess the S.O.B.—an elderly rancher with emphysema. Took his history, asked all the pertinent questions. Listened to his lungs, his heart, called for a chest X-ray. His wife was with him, silver-haired and gnarled as an old tree branch, likely just as tough.

"Have a seat, Ma'am. Doc Halliday will be in as soon as she is able."

Going back to the trauma room, I found the team had Stormy intubated, stabilized and was preparing to send her to surgery. Doc suspected a ruptured spleen and other internal injuries. Sinus tach at a rate of 118, blood pressure 90 over 62. The room was trashed, but the patient, alive. I felt a small sense of satisfaction. And something else. Gratitude, maybe?

O.R. sent their own people down to transport Stormy to Surgery. They showed up unannounced, in their green scrubs and booties, bonnets over their Stetsons, and surgical masks covering their mustachios. Not bothering to wait for report, they wheel her away.

I looked around the room, it's trashed like only a trauma room after a code can be. Oh, but wait—they forgot her patient belonging bag. The only thing inside it was the one tassel, all she had on when she arrived, but it was her tittie tassel, just the same. I wrote her name *Stormy Wether* in a black marker on the outside of the bag.

"Will you cover for me?" I asked Tonto who came in to help me clean up the room. "I'm going to run this to Surgery."

"Wait, Carson," Doc Halliday said, handing me a printout. "Take these lab results up too, please. They just came through."

"Go on, Kit, I've got your back," Tonto said.

"Where *is* Surgery?" I asked, feeling stupid. I had never been beyond Wellmart's Emergency Department.

"Basement," Halliday barked, leaving the room to see to the next patient.

"Underground, level two," she said over her shoulder.

Snatching up the plastic bag, I hurried to catch up with the patient. She should have a nurse in attendance. Down the hallway, I saw the surgery techs inside the elevator, the gurney with Stormy Wether between them. I could hear the monitor beeping.

"Wait!" I called to them, but the elevator door closed.

I made for the stairwell, skipping steps, thinking to catch them when they got off the lift two floors below. I didn't count stepping on something—a needle cap? a pen? a bullet casing? Whatever it was, it rolled under my boot and I did a little hoedown trying to keep my footing but ended up falling, twisting my ankle as I went down hard. A sharp pain told me it was probably sprained. Damn! Gingerly, I pulled my foot out of the boot and sure enough, the ankle was already swelling. Responding quickly, I wrapped it with surgical tape—I always carry a roll of it on hemostats clipped to my scrub top. I'm nothing, if not prepared. Then I put my boot back on and hobbled the rest of the way down to Level II Underground.

The elevator was empty. Damn.

I followed the signs to Surgery, limping along like Hopalong Cassidy. My ankle was shooting sparks, but I gritted my teeth and kept going. Outside of the double doors marked

Surgery

I mashed on the automatic opener—but nothing happened. Pulled out my phone to call them—but there was no signal down here. I knocked on the door and heard the intercom crackle.

"Surgery. State your business."

"I'm Kit Carson from the ER. I've got belongings for the patient we just sent you."

The doors swung open to allow me in. A young male clerk behind the desk looked at me curiously.

"From Emergency, are you? Well, that's great, but where's the famous pole dancer? I hear we're about to get a little stormy weather down here."

"She isn't here?" I said, ignoring his innuendos. "That's impossible. I saw her in the elevator two minutes ago. She should be here by now."

"Sounds to me like you lost your patient, Nurse Carson."

"But your people from Surgery came and got her. I was there, I saw them."

"You're mistaken, pardner. We didn't send anybody. We're understaffed; it's just the on-call team here." He grinned. "I think you better go find that stripper. Our guys are scrubbed and ready."

Confused, I turned to leave, still clutching the bag with Stormy's tassel in it. Seeing a wheelchair by the door, I plopped down in the seat.

"Borrowing this rig," I said.

The clerk shrugged. "Ride 'em cowgirl." He turned back to his work.

"Hi ho Silver." I spun the wheelchair around and wheeled out. Which way should I go? Where could they have gone?

Hospital basements are creepy, especially late at night. They might be your best bet in a tornado, but without windows or doors to the outside world it was gloomy as the catacombs down here. All the heavy emotions felt throughout the hospital—fear, pain, grief—have to go somewhere. Maybe they sink like cold air. I could feel them now, a damp cloud; a miasma of sadness.

Halfway down the long corridor, I stopped, got my phone out and tried to call Tonto, but I didn't have a signal down here in the transverse colon of Wellmart's bowels. Seeing a few dots on the waxed hallway floor, I leaned over in the chair for a better look. Blood. Fresh blood, not quite dry. I rolled along, found some more. A trail of blood leading me where? Whose blood? Stormy's? That didn't make sense. She wasn't bleeding except internally. Whose blood?

The trail stopped at the end of the hall. There were two doors on either side. One said

Engineering

From within I could hear the low rumbling hum of the machinery; I could feel the vibration in my bones. I looked through the window. It was dark inside and the door was locked.

The door across the hall was a solid, windowless door with weather sealing. A plaque on the wall next to it said:

Pathology Cold Storage

No Admittance except authorized personnel

Deeming myself authorized, I turned the handle and to my surprise the door opened easily. I rolled the wheelchair inside. It was icy cold and smelled of formaldehyde.

Feeling uneasy, I drew my gun from the holster and released the safety. Thought I heard a scuttling. Rats? It was a lab so maybe there were lab rats. Maybe they did testing or experiments down here.

I felt around and found the light switch on the wall behind me. Florescent overheads whined, flickered erratically a few times, then went out altogether. Must be a bad ballast, I thought. But there should be more lights somewhere. Propping the door open with the wheelchair, I got up, walking slowly on my ankle, wincing from the pain. Found my pocket penlight and looked around at what appeared to be a large storage room. Kind of cluttered, for a lab. It looked more like a storage room, with unused equipment stacked against the wall—sterilizers, autoclaves, centrifuges, coolers. Boxes of petri dishes, solvents, stains, and cell culture media. On the bench, trays of scalpels and disposable knives laid out. I picked one up and pocketed it; they're handy to have.

Heard a muffled sound, a scuffling, and a little squeak from the rodents. They're active at night, I've heard. Or maybe they were complaining of the cold; it felt like a damn refrigerator in here.

I switched the light off, put it back in my pocket. Now holding my gun in both hands, I looked around me, hyperaware, casing the room like they do in the movies.

I inched my way deeper into the dark space, my ankle protesting with every step. I shivered, but was it from the cold or from fear? A few steps more...

My eyes began to adjust to the dark. Just ahead, gurneys – a row of them, like horses tied to the hitching post. Six, to be exact. I hobbled closer, my stomach tightening and the hair on my arms standing up as I realized where I was. The gurneys had bodies on them. This was the cold storage holding area for Wellmart's dead patients. I was in the hospital morgue.

Even with her face covered by a sheet, I recognized Stormy by her breasts, still pointing skyward, firm and proud as the Grand Tetons. With one hand I yanked back the sheet to see her face, drained of all color except for her permanently tattooed lips, resplendently red. I refused to believe she was dead – she had been transported out of the ER alive and stable only five minutes ago. Reflexively, I shook her shoulder, cold but not stiff.

"Stormy!" I hissed.

Stormy did not respond. I leaned close and turned my head, listening and feeling for breath on my cheek, but my own face was numb from the cold. Laying my gun down next to her head, I opened her airway with a jaw thrust, pinched off her nose and delivered two breaths, my lips covering hers, watching her chest rise and fall, rise and fall. Then I felt for a carotid pulse. The portable heart monitor had been turned off, but it was still sitting between her ankles at the foot of the cart. There was an IV pole and the bag of normal saline was still dripping into her vein. What the fuck? Who did this? Ratzer's men?

Balmy had been right, of course. They were here in the hospital. It must have been them behind the surgical masks. Maybe they had Balmy.

Just then I heard the squeaking sound, louder. I sucked in my breath as the corpse on the next gurney writhed under the sheet. Pushing Stormy's gurney aside, I went to the moving corpse, flung off the sheet and found Balmy, gagged and bound to the side rail. With my trusty bandage scissors, I cut the tape across her mouth. She spit out a wad of gauze and gasped for breath.

"Look out! He's got my knife!"

I never even saw him. If I had, or if I had sensed his presence, I might have throat-chopped him or smashed his balls with an awesome kickbox move. Too late, I ducked—but the assailant had me by the hair, yanked me up against him, the cold steel blade pressing against my neck. Instinctively, I froze, not daring to breathe. Too late, my martial arts training kicked in. *Feign submission. Distract opponent.*

"Please, mister, call the doctor," I whispered, sinking against his bulk, raising my arms in a gesture of surrender, then anticipating a momentary shift in his attention, I grabbed his wrist at my neck—the thick, hairy wrist—pulling it down against my chest, rotating the blade outward. Next I tried to pivot under the assailant's arm, like Master Bunn taught us, but it wasn't happening. This thug had me smashed against the gurney with his bulk, I wasn't going anywhere. So I chomped down on his arm like I was biting into an ear of corn, and he dropped the knife alright, but the next thing I knew I was on the floor and this fat fucking ox was on top of me. I couldn't breathe. Why had I stopped jiujitsu after earning a white belt? I cursed myself for being such a dilettante, for not following through with anything. Except nursing. I'm a good nurse, a damn good nurse.

I remembered, with dismay and remorse, my weapon. I hadn't put the pistol back in my holster, but instead, had laid it on gurney when I tried to revive Stormy – for the second time that night. You can't be a good nurse with a gun in your hand.

I could hear the rattle of the side rails as Balmy, still bound, struggled against a second attacker. "No!" she blurted out, followed by muffled curses and grunts.

In desperation, I tried to scream but it came out a whisper. I couldn't breathe. Like a mule, I drew my knees up and kicked out, trying to buck him off. If only I could get off my back and onto my side, if only I could breathe! I fought the wave of panic crashing over me.

Wait until he makes his next move, I heard Master Bunn say calmly in my mind. I prepared myself to take advantage of the any change. I knew I had to be quick and sure. Sure enough, he shifted his weight to grab my wrists, and as soon as he did, I pulled my arms in close to my body, twisting my torso to one side. My arms were now free, but he swung, his fist hitting the side of my face. My ears rang, darkness closed in, and I fought to stay conscious.

"Drop it!"

It was Halliday's voice, was I imagining it?

"Right now, you sons-a-bitches." She stood in the doorway, backlit by the lights from the corridor. Guns drawn, slouch hat pulled low over her brow, stethoscope looped around her neck. For a long moment no one moved.

Then came the snap crackle of pistol fire from the goon by Balmy and Halliday stumbled back, clutching her shoulder, collapsing into a stack of crates. It all went down with a crash of breaking glass.

I felt the man on top of me move; I drew in a breath and struggled to get up, but his hand slammed my head back against the floor. The room seemed to tilt and whirl. Sparks rained down behind my eyes; shooting stars, like arrows, fell out of the sky. I thought I saw Tonto's face above me, up in the clouds. It was Tonto's face, yes, but streaked with war paint. Was I dying?

I fought against the delirium, struggled to stay awake. Heard a chilling, unearthly war cry pierce the air, then *Thwop Thwop.* The man on top of me slumped over like he was suddenly exhausted. I heard the last breath leave his body in a sigh. Squirming to get out from under him, I felt his hot, spurting blood and saw a well-placed arrow deep in the side of his neck. The other attacker was face down on top of Balmy, an arrow shaft sticking out of his cervical spine.

Tonto looked down from the duct space overhead, a ceiling tile removed. He hung from a pipe, then dropped down soft as a cat in his moccasins, bow in hand. His torso was bare and hairless; a quiver strapped to his back. He knelt over me, his dark eyes peering into mine.

"I'm alive," I panted. "Balmy. Help her. Halliday's been hit."

"I'm able," Doc said as she staggered through the broken beakers and petri dishes, gripping her left shoulder. "It's only a scratch." She made her way to Stormy's side, feeling for a pulse; I struggled to my feet, head ringing, to assist.

Tonto freed Balmy from her restraints and left her assailant in her place on the gurney, covering him with the blood-stained sheet. Just then the dancer stirred and mumbled, "Will somebody bring me a goddamn blanket? It's freezing in here!"

*

We rushed Stormy up to the chopper pad, where a chopper was waiting. Halliday had called for an emergency air transport for Stormy (under the alias of Nellie Smith) to Dodge City Trauma Center, beyond Ratzer's reach. For the moment, she

33

was safe. But we had our work cut out for us, to expose the sheriff and bring him to justice. The dead men we left in the morgue, a coroner's case that would either be investigated or covered up, depending on Razer's influence.

Back in the ER, we patched up Halliday's wound before the day shift started to straggle in. She was lucky; the bullet had missed both artery and bone.

*

07:30.

Tonto walked us to my ride, parked in the North Forty. Clearly the law in this town could not be trusted; Balmy had to lay low until Ratzer was exposed. She was to bunk up with me and the kids until she could be reunited with her sister in Dodge City. In the meanwhile, I figured she could babysit my kids and study for her G.E.D.

"I want to keep an eye on you," Tonto said. "We can't be too careful. Don't know how many men Ratzer has working for him."

I told him where I lived.

*

I cancelled my shift that evening; my ankle was swollen like a fence post. Scrounged the cupboards, found a single can of pork and beans for Wyatt, Cassidy, and Balmy to share for supper. I collapsed in front of the television to binge on

Smokin' Guns, Season Three on DVD, the cable having been shut off last week. But the throaty rumble of a motorcycle interrupted my plan.

"It's the Indian," Balmy said, peering out the window. "He's here."

The engine stopped, and a moment later the doorbell rang.

"Let him in," I said, my heart knocking.

What luck, I thought. Tim Rhodes standing in my living room in his bike leathers—with Chinese take-out, a six pack of beer, and a bundle of sage under his arm.

"I just stopped by to make sure you all were safe. Thought you'd want to know, I spoke with Doc Halliday. Stormy reached Dodge City safely and just got out of surgery. A successful splenectomy. She's in stable condition."

After Tonto saged us and cleansed the room, we all sat cross-legged on the floor, our laps for a table, feasting on Happy Family, beef and broccoli, noodles and rice from Hop Sing's Kitchen. Balmy soon fell asleep on the couch, fast and hard like only a teenager can. Tonto played a few hands of Faro with Wyatt and Cassidy while I took a hot bath. Then it was bedtime for the kids. Tonto took his leave, putting on his leather jacket and goggles.

"Good night, Kemosabe. Get some sleep, I'll call you tomorrow."

I watched through the window as he drove his motorcycle into the moonrise. Tucked the kids in, turned the lights out, covered Balmy with a spare blanket. Only then did I eat my fortune cookie, saving the message until I had swallowed the last crumb.

∞

To be continued...

Sunday Night Knife & Gun Club

Episode #3 of Nurse Kit Carson's Adventures

by L.S. Collison

ISBN: 978-1-7322290-2-0 (paperback)
ISBN: 978-1-7322290-1-3 (electronic)